The need to
nutrition ı

How your food and drink can help you to achieve
your workout goals

By

Tim Shaw BSc MSc

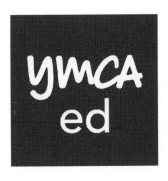

*Discover more books and ebooks of interest to you and find out about the range
of work we do at the forefront of health, fitness and wellbeing.*

www.ymcaed.org.uk

Published by Central YMCA Trading Ltd (trading as YMCAed).
Registered Company No. 3667206.

YMCAed
Central YMCA Trading Ltd
112 Great Russell Street
London
WC1B 3NQ

www.ymcaed.org.uk

This book is presented solely for educational and entertainment purposes. The author and publisher are not offering it as legal, medical, or other professional services advice. While best efforts have been used in preparing this book, the author and publisher make no representations or warranties of any kind and assume no liabilities of any kind with respect to the accuracy or completeness of the contents and specifically disclaim any implied warranties of merchantability or fitness of use for a particular purpose. Neither the publisher nor the individual author(s) shall be liable for any physical, psychological, emotional, financial, or commercial damages, including, but not limited to, special, incidental, consequential or other damages, resulting from the information or programs contained herein. Every person is different and the information, advice and programs contained herein may not be suitable for your situation. Exercise is not without its risks and, as such, we would strongly advise that you consult with your healthcare professional before beginning any programme of exercise, especially if you have, or suspect you may have, any injuries or illnesses, are currently pregnant or have recently given birth. The advice, information and guidance given in Central YMCA Guides is in no way intended as a substitute for medical consultation. As with any form of exercise, you should stop immediately if you feel faint, dizzy or have physical discomfort or pain or any other contra indication, and consult a physician.

Central YMCA is the world's founding YMCA. Established in 1844 in Central London, it was the first YMCA to open its doors and, in so doing, launched a movement that has now grown to become the world's biggest youth organisation. Today, Central YMCA is the UK's leading health, fitness and wellbeing charity, committed to helping people from all walks of life – and specifically the young and those with a specific need – to live happier, healthier and more fulfilled lives.

CONTENTS

ABOUT THE AUTHOR

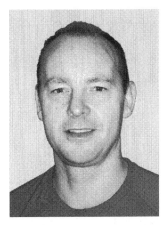

Hello and thanks for reading this book.

I am an experienced instructor in the health and fitness industry, specialising in teaching the principles of exercise, nutrition and healthy eating to gym instructors and personal trainers. I am also involved in teaching fitness for disabled clients and training for older adults.

I have worked for London Central YMCA as a tutor in health and fitness for over 20 years. Prior to that I studied engineering and have a BSc in technology and an MSc in robotics.

My interest in nutrition first began back in the 1980s and over the past three decades I have tried most diets and food fads for myself, ultimately concluding that they are largely unnecessary and that the best nutrition is actually achieved by following simple guidelines and eating the right balance of healthy foods.

My first book – 'The need to know guide to nutrition and healthy eating' (ymcaed.org.uk/nahe) – took a back to basics look at food and drink and the steps we all need to take to ensure we are eating and drinking healthily for our bodies. This book, however, takes things further and looks specifically at nutrition for exercise. It is aimed at those of you who enjoy exercise and who are aware of, or at least interested in, how the food and drink you consume can affect how you exercise.

I hope you enjoy the book.

Tim

INTRODUCTION

If you are an active person who exercises regularly in order to stay fit, then this guide is for you. Good nutrition is an essential part of getting the most out of any exercise. You can follow the best training programme, but without the right types of food at the right times and in the right quantities for your body, you will not make optimum progress.

Good nutrition can help with several key aspects of exercise. These include:

1. Having energy to train without fatigue
2. Staying hydrated
3. Promoting recovery after an exercise session
4. Maintaining an optimum body weight
5. Reducing the stress on your immune system caused by training

If you are a more serious athlete who likes to compete, there can be other benefits too, including:

1. Building muscle size, strength and power
2. Optimising performance for long-distance events like a triathlon or marathon

The primary philosophy is to follow a diet based around a balanced intake of healthy foods. Over the course of this book we will look at healthy eating guidelines, and then at how these will need to be modified for active people. Common themes include: the increased need for energy, carbohydrates and proteins, the importance of hydration, limiting intake of fats to healthy sources, and increasing fruit and vegetable intake to meet greater micronutrient demands. We will also explore some of the most commonly available supplements, and discuss how their judicious use can enhance performance.

Compared to healthy eating, nutrition for exercise requires a little more technical detail to obtain optimum results. So, be warned: you will be encountering formulae, grams, calories and percentages over the following pages.

1

GETTING THE BALANCE RIGHT

Most countries use some form of the 'healthy eating plate' with food groups and portion numbers to describe how we should eat for the benefit of our health. Each country's guidelines are slightly different, but the basic message can be summarised as follows:

Food group	Recommended portions/day	What is a portion?
Complex carbohydrates	6 – 11	1 slice of bread, 1 small bread roll, 1 potato, ½ cup of cooked rice or pasta, 30g (just over 1oz) breakfast cereal, etc.
Fruit and vegetables	5 – 9	1 medium fruit (apple, orange, banana, etc.), handful of berries or grapes, one 125ml (5fl oz) glass fruit juice or smoothie, 1 small bowl of salad, ½ cup of cooked vegetables.
Protein-rich foods	2 – 3	Meat, fish, chicken, tofu (size of a deck of cards), 1 egg, ½ cup of cooked beans or pulses, etc.
Dairy foods	2 – 3	1 small carton of yoghurt, one 200ml (⅓ pint) glass of milk, 40g (nearly 2oz) cheese – size of a small matchbox.
Healthy fats	2 – 3	2 teaspoons of olive oil, oily fish (size of a deck of cards), ½ an avocado, 2 tablespoons of nuts or seeds, etc.
Foods high in unhealthy fats and refined sugar	0 – 1 (eat sparingly)	1 biscuit, 1 slice of cake, 1 can of soft drink, 25g (1oz) bag of crisps, 1 small bowl of chocolate pudding, 125ml glass fruit juice or smoothie (if you have more than 1 per day), etc.

(Bean, 2003) (www.dh.gov.uk, 2012) (www.choosemyplate.gov, 2012) (www.hsph.harvard.edu, 2012)

However, these portion numbers are more suited to sedentary people than active people, so when it comes to nutrition for exercise these guidelines may not be sufficient.

If you exercise regularly, then you can benefit from adjusting your diet somewhat from this standard model. In particular, your intake of complex carbs, fruit and vegetables will all increase. Portions of protein-rich foods and dairy foods will also increase, but with a focus on lower fat versions. Portions of healthy fats either stay the same or increase slightly. Thus the calories from fat, as a percentage of the whole, actually decrease. Unhealthy fats still remain the 'bad guys' in the performance diet and portions eaten should be kept to a minimum. But, as we shall see, the guidelines for refined sugars become more ambiguous because they may play a significant role in rapid refuelling during and after training.

The pie charts that follow represent total calories consumed per day, and how those calories are divided between fats, proteins and carbohydrates. The first chart shows typical proportions for healthy eating. The second shows how this adjusts to supply the demands of an active lifestyle.

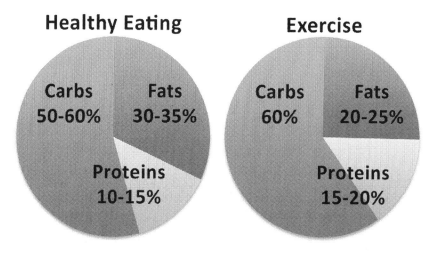

Notice that the Exercise chart is considerably larger than the first, reflecting the increased overall energy intake for someone who exercises. Notice also that the proportions of carbs and protein intakes both increase, whilst fat intake becomes more restricted.

Clearly some details will change depending upon whether you are more of a weight trainer interested in building strength and muscle mass, or whether you prefer endurance training and like to participate in aerobics, running, triathlon, etc. But if you get bogged down in any of the detail or conflicting arguments in the following chapters, it is good to have the basic concepts of food groups, portion numbers, and percentages of fats, proteins and carbs to refer back to.

KEEPING TRACK OF WHAT YOU EAT

You will need some means of keeping track of your diet so you can check if you are meeting your nutrition guidelines.

One practical idea is to use a table to record the portions of each food group you eat on a daily basis. The table is blank at the start of the day, and you simply add a mark whenever you consume a portion of that particular food group. At the end of the day you can total each column to see how close you are to your target portions. For example:

Foods group	Complex carbohydrates	Fruit and vegetables	Protein-rich foods	Dairy	Healthy fats	Foods high in unhealthy fats and refined sugar
Portions eaten	IIIII III Total = 8	II Total = 2	III Total = 3	III Total = 3	I Total = 1	IIIII II Total = 7

In this example the intake of fruit and veg clearly needs to increase, and the quantity of foods high in processed fats and sugars is much too high. So it is easy to identify how eating can be improved the next day. Improvements can be made gradually. In this case, a good start would be to decline some of the fatty, sugary snacks and replace them with some fruit instead.

An alternative approach is to record each food you eat in detail, making a note of the grams of fats, proteins and carbs. This takes more time and effort than recording portions, but it can yield more useful results. You will need to study nutrition labels of the products you eat to get accurate figures. If you eat cereal, rice, pasta etc., then it is best to weigh them out to be sure exactly how much you are eating. Information can be recorded in a food diary, like this:

Food	Fat (g)	Protein (g)	Carb (g)
60g cornflakes	0.5	4	52
250ml semi-skimmed milk	6.5	10	15
Omelette (3 eggs)	18	21	0
Chips (medium portion)	19	4	38
250ml orange juice	0	0	31
Etc.			

At the end of a day's eating the grams in each column can be totalled, then the total energy consumed and percentages obtained from fats, proteins and carbs can be calculated.

Note that 1g fat contains 9kcal, 1g protein contains 4kcal and 1g carbohydrate contains 4kcal. For example:

	Fat (g)	Protein (g)	Carbs (g)
Totals (g)	92	122	301
Kcal	(x9) = 828	(x4) = 488	(x4) = 1,204
Total kcal	828 + 488 + 1204 = 2,520		
Kcal as a percentage of total	828/2,520 = 33%	488/2,520 = 19%	1,204/2,520 = 48%

So in this example, 2,520kcal in total were eaten. This figure can be compared to energy requirements (see next chapter). We also see that too many calories come from fat (33% compared to the recommended 20 – 25%), whilst the diet is deficient in carbs (48% not 60%). Protein intake is 19% which falls comfortably within the 15 – 20% recommended range. (Bean, 2003).

If you don't like the idea of writing down this information and performing these calculations every day, there are websites and smartphone apps to help you complete this type of analysis.

2

ENERGY REQUIREMENTS

The first step in planning a diet for exercise is to calculate how much energy you need each day. There are two parts to the calculation: The first gives your basal metabolic rate (BMR) which is the sum of all the energy used in 24 hours to stay alive and maintain basic metabolic processes such as bodily warmth, breathing, circulation and cellular function. The second part estimates your activity level using a physical activity factor (PAF):

PART 1: BASAL METABOLIC RATE (BMR)

BMR is mainly dependent on your age, gender and body weight. To calculate this we will use the Schofield equation (Schofield, 1985):

Women
10 – 17 years:	BMR = 13.4 x W + 692
18 – 29 years:	BMR = 14.8 x W + 487
30 – 59 years:	BMR = 8.3 x W + 846

Men
10 – 17 years:	BMR = 17.7 x W + 657
18 – 29 years:	BMR = 15.1 x W + 692
30 – 59 years:	BMR = 11.5 x W + 873

(W = body weight in kilograms)

For example:

Judy, a 49-year-old female weighing 62kg, has a BMR of: 8.3 x 62 + 846 = 1,360.6kcal

Jack, a 23-year-old male weighing 85kg, has a BMR of: 15.1 x 85 + 692 = 1,975.5kcal

The BMR figure tells us the minimum calories needed for the body to maintain itself for 24 hours, before any activity is done.

PART 2: PHYSICAL ACTIVITY FACTOR (PAF)

Multiply the figure from part 1 by the PAF, depending on whether the person is inactive, moderately active or very active:

		PAF Women	PAF Men
Inactive	Desk job, drive everywhere or take public transport, negligible exercise or active pastimes	1.4	1.4
Moderately active	Moderately active job involving standing, walking, etc. Regular 3 x weekly gym visits or playing social sports	1.6	1.7
Very active	Very active job involving lifting and carrying, etc. Regular 5 x weekly gym visits with intense, longer duration training sessions or playing intense, competitive sports	1.8	1.9

So if Judy is very active, her PAF is 1.8 and her daily kcal total is:

1360.6 x 1.8 = 2,449kcal

If Jack is very active, his PAF is 1.9 and his daily kcal total is:

1975.5 x 1.9 = 3,753kcal

The daily kcal total can then be used to calculate how much fat, protein and carbohydrate should be eaten. For example:

Judy: Fats   2,449 x 25% = 612kcal   612/9 = 68g fats
          Proteins   2,449 x 15% = 367kcal   367/4 = 92g proteins
          Carbs   2,449 x 60% = 1,470kcal   1,470/4 = 368g carbs

Jack: Fats   3,753 x 25% = 938kcal   938/9 = 104g fats
          Proteins   3,753 x 15% = 563kcal   563/4 = 141g proteins
          Carbs   3,753 x 60% = 2,252kcal   2,252/4 = 563g carbs

You then have all the information you need to analyse a detailed food diary. (Note: Figures of 25% fats and 15% proteins used as an illustration. Figures anywhere within ranges shown in the pie chart can be used according to your needs.)

Clearly any method like this makes a number of assumptions and is therefore subject to error, but for most purposes it is accurate enough. It is possible, with the use of some technology, to make a direct measurement of how much energy you expend in a day. For example, if you perform a regular workout on a treadmill, then the calorie count is displayed. Check that you enter your body weight for the figure to be accurate. If you want to spend money, then electronic devices are available that combine heart rate monitoring with accelerometer technology to give an accurate measurement of daily energy used.

WHAT HAPPENS IF MY ENERGY INTAKE IS TOO HIGH?

If you consume too many calories then you will gain weight. This can be good or bad depending upon your aims. If you want to gain lean muscle then eating calories over and above your maintenance level is essential. Of course the excess energy must be combined with intense resistance training for weight gain to be in the form of lean muscle (chapter 9). If you just eat too much and don't exercise then the weight gain will be in the form of body fat.

WHAT HAPPENS IF MY ENERGY INTAKE IS TOO LOW?

If you consume too few calories for your needs then you will lose weight. This can also be either good or bad depending upon your goals. If you are aiming to lose body fat then calorie restriction is a necessary part of your programme, but it needs to be within certain limits to ensure healthy fat loss over time. If you restrict calorie intake too severely and also want to maintain an exercise programme, then there are other risks you need to consider. Something called 'energy availability' can be a useful measure to ensure you eat enough calories to avoid major health problems.

ENERGY AVAILABILITY

The concept of energy availability is quite recent (Loucks, Kiens, & Wright, 2011). Essentially, it is a method of checking that your body has enough energy available to remain healthy once all the energy for exercise has been considered.

Energy availability = energy intake – energy for training and exercise

There appears to be a threshold energy intake of about 30kcal per kg of fat free mass (FFM) needed to avoid problems such as reduced immunity, menstrual disturbances, decreased bone density and impaired hormone function.

Fat free mass is your body mass minus fat mass. To calculate this you will need to know your body fat percentage. This can be estimated easily using a digital 'bioelectrical impedance' device, or using body fat callipers. Ask at your gym.

Using our previous example, if Judy, our 62kg female, has a body fat percentage of 20%, then her fat mass is:

62 x 20% = 12.4kg

Therefore her fat free mass (what remains if all her fat is removed) is:

62 – 12.4 = 49.6kg

So, once energy for exercise has been considered, her energy availability is:

49.6 x 30kcal = 1,488kcal

In other words, this is the basic minimum energy her body needs each day to remain healthy.

For Jack, if his body fat is 14%, the calculation is:

Fat mass: 85 x 14% = 11.9kg

Fat free mass: 85 – 11.9 = 73.1kg

Energy availability: 73.1 x 30kcal = 2,193kcal

These figures are a little higher than the BMR figures from the Schofield calculation. This makes sense assuming our example people are more active than average and therefore have more metabolically active muscle than the typical sedentary individual. Thus, energy availability is another useful check to make sure you are eating enough calories to remain healthy.

HOW MUCH ENERGY IS STORED AS FAT?

We have just calculated that Judy has 12.4kg of body fat. To convert this into energy we simply use the conversion: 1g fat = 9kcal (or 1kg fat = 9,000kcal), therefore 12.4kg of body fat at 9,000kcal per kg equals a total of 111,600kcal of stored energy. True, some of this is 'essential fat' forming part of the central nervous system, insulating nerves, cushioning joints, etc. Also, the conversion from stored fat to useful energy for muscular work is not 100% efficient, typically reducing the availability to around 7,000kcal per kg. This gives a realistic figure of about 80,000kcal of energy stored as fat. Even so, this is a huge fuel tank and unlikely to run out, even in an ultra-distance race lasting for several days. Calculated in similar fashion, Jack has about 75,000kcal of energy stored as fat.

HOW DOES THE BODY USE FOOD TO PRODUCE ENERGY?

Your body has three metabolic pathways or 'energy systems' to create energy for exercise. They can all be active at any given moment to a greater or lesser extent, depending primarily on the intensity of the activity.

System 1: Exercise that is moderate intensity and continuous in nature, such as walking, jogging, cycling or swimming, uses the aerobic pathway. This can be fuelled by a mix of fats (from stored body fat), carbohydrates (from stored glycogen) and proteins (from the breakdown of muscles). Aerobic energy production has no limit to duration so long as you have those fuels available and you are breathing to deliver oxygen to the muscles and clear away carbon dioxide.

System 2: Exercise that is high intensity, such as interval training, weight training or circuit training, uses the anaerobic pathway fuelled exclusively by carbohydrates in the form of stored glycogen. This is known as anaerobic glycolysis. It can only last for a limited time of around 60 – 90 seconds because a by-product called lactic acid (lactate and H^+ ions) accumulates in the muscles, causing the familiar burning/aching sensation and preventing further activity until you stop, rest and recover.

System 3: Exercise of 'explosive' intensity, such as sprinting, Olympic weight lifting, power lifting, jumping and throwing uses another anaerobic pathway. Here, a cellular chemical in the muscles called creatine phosphate provides a source of instant energy. But muscular stores are only good enough for about 6 – 10 seconds of maximal effort before they are depleted. Once depleted, full recovery is needed to allow the muscles to replenish muscular stores of creatine phosphate. Within 20 seconds, approximately 50% is replenished. After 40 seconds, around 75% is replenished, and so on, meaning that 3 – 4 minutes are required for most of the creatine phosphate to have replenished, ready for a further burst of maximal effort (Fleck & Kraemer, 1987).

It is logical to think that if you could increase your muscular stores of creatine phosphate then you could perform a greater volume of maximal exercise, and indeed this does seem to be the case. Hence the prevalence of creatine supplements (see Chapter 8).

The three energy pathways are summarised in the following table:

Energy pathway	Exercise Duration	Exercise Intensity	Example activities	Fuel(s)
Aerobic	On-going	Low – moderate	Walk Jog Swim Cycle	Fats Carbs (glycogen) Proteins
Anaerobic glycolysis	60 – 90 seconds (After this time the accumulation of lactate/H^+ ions in blood prevents further muscle contraction)	High	Weight training Circuit training Interval training	Carbs (glycogen)
Creatine phosphate	6 – 10 seconds (after this time the muscular stores of creatine phosphate become depleted)	Very High	Sprinting Weight lifting Power lifting Jumping Throwing	Creatine phosphate

There are some important lessons to be learned from the three energy pathways and applied to exercise nutrition. Firstly, carbohydrates in the form of stored glycogen are used no matter what type of training you do. Whether it is low intensity jogging, weight training or high intensity intervals, you must have enough glycogen in your muscles for energy to train. Then, after training, it is equally important to replenish those glycogen stores ready for the next workout. This will be a recurring theme in the following pages.

Secondly, fat is used directly as a fuel only for aerobic exercise at low-to-moderate intensity. Fat cannot be used in the absence of oxygen and therefore does not fuel anaerobic exercise. Fat is the long-term fuel supply for your metabolic needs, plus all your day-to-day activities like standing, walking, housework, etc. Interestingly, one of the many benefits of cardiovascular training is that your muscles become better at utilising fat and sparing glycogen.

Although anaerobic exercise like weight training does not directly burn fat it still has a significant role in controlling body fat by maintaining lean muscle and hence maintaining a higher metabolic rate.

The third significant point is that proteins can be used for energy. This is not something the body favours because proteins are so important for repair and maintenance. However, if glycogen stores are low and energy is still needed (e.g. in the last few kilometres of a marathon) then protein becomes the only option. Your body does not have a 'store' of protein in the same way that it does of carbs (glycogen) or fats (adipose tissue). Instead it must obtain protein by breaking down your muscles, organs and other tissues. This 'cannibalising' of your own body is something to be avoided as much as possible. The main key to preventing this is to eat sufficient amounts of carbohydrate.

3

CARBOHYDRATES

From the previous chapter it is clear that carbs are essential as the main fuel for exercise. Whether you like cardiovascular training such as running, cycling, swimming or aerobics classes, or you mainly train with weights, you will always use carbs to power your workout.

HOW ARE CARBOHYDRATES DIGESTED AND STORED?

Carbs are eaten either as starches (complex) or sugars (simple). Once digested, all carbohydrates enter the blood in the form of glucose. If you have eaten a meal with large serving of carbs then more glucose will enter the blood than you need at that moment. As glucose levels ('blood sugar levels') rise, your pancreas releases the hormone insulin which, in turn, transports the excess glucose into storage in your liver and muscles as glycogen.

Glycogen is the stored form of carbohydrate in the body and it is essential for fuelling any exercise you do.

The liver can store about 70 – 100g glycogen, whilst the muscles can store about 100 – 300g of glycogen, depending upon your body size. This gives between to 170 – 400g in total, which equates to around 680 – 1,600kcal of energy stored as glycogen (Cahill, 1976) (Wootton, 1990). This may seem sufficient, but in reality only a proportion of this total glycogen store is actually available for exercise. Firstly, much of the liver glycogen is there to fuel the central nervous system, not for exercise. Secondly, muscle glycogen usage is specific to the muscle where it is stored. If you run, glycogen stored in the hip and leg muscles is used. If you complete a set of biceps curls, then just the glycogen in your biceps is used. So even though total glycogen storage may be enough, it is not necessarily in the muscles where you need it at that particular instant.

Compare this to the energy stored in body fat. In Chapter 2 our example people had somewhere in the region of 75 – 80,000kcal of fat available to fuel exercise, which is at least *fifty* times the glycogen available.

HOW MUCH CARBOHYDRATE SHOULD I EAT?

Glycogen is used up when you exercise and it is replaced by eating carbs. It is not replenished to any significant extent by eating fats or proteins or by drinking alcohol. This is important to understand. You can be taking in sufficient total calories, but if the proportions of fats, proteins and carbohydrates are wrong, you will not have the optimum muscle fuel to train and you will feel fatigued more quickly. So eating carbs is crucial.

There is a limit to how fast glycogen can be replenished. Typically, after an intense training session, muscle stores take between 24 – 48 hours to replenish fully (Coyle, 1995). This is one of the reasons why one to two days' recovery time is recommended between intense workouts. The continual replenishment process over a number of hours implies that each meal and snack eaten should include carbs. In other words, they form a basis for a high-energy training diet (Coyle, 1991). Endurance athletes should maintain a consistently high carbohydrate intake to replenish glycogen stores (60% of total kcal).

The post-training meal is of particular importance. This is because the body is in a state of stress immediately following hard exercise, with an increased demand for nutrients to facilitate the recovery process. The muscles' ability to replenish glycogen is greatest in the first two hours or so right after exercise. Eating carbohydrates stimulates insulin release, which in turn facilitates the transport of glucose from the blood into storage as muscle glycogen. In other words, just the right conditions exist for glycogen to be replenished quickly. Ingesting quickly absorbed carbs immediately after training also reduces post-training levels of cortisol, a stress hormone related to suppression of the immune system (Tarpenning, 2001).

Researchers recommend you eat 1g carbohydrate for every kg body weight in the two hours immediately following training (Bean, 2003). Using our example people from Chapter 2, Judy would need to eat 62g carbs and Jack would aim for 85g carbs. In real world terms, this quantity of carbs could be provided by any of the following:

- [ ] 3 – 4 slices of bread
- [ ] 80 – 100g breakfast cereal
- [ ] 200 – 250g of cooked pasta
- [ ] 500 – 750ml bottle of energy drink
- [ ] 1 medium – large cola from a fast food restaurant

These examples are not a recommendation; they simply show that there is a wide choice about the type and quality of the carbs you could consume. This depends partly on convenience and personal preference, but also on speed of absorption. Contrary to healthy eating guidelines, there is a strong argument for using fast-acting high GI carbs immediately following a training session.

WHICH IS BEST: LOW OR HIGH GI?

The glycaemic index, or GI, is a measure of how quickly different types of carbohydrates elevate blood glucose levels. A glucose drink is used as the reference food (GI = 100) and then other foods are compared to this reference point and given a number on a 1 – 100 scale.

High GI carbs such as a refined breakfast cereal (GI = 80+) will raise blood sugar significantly within minutes of ingestion. Lower GI carbs such as those found in apples (GI = 38) or porridge (GI = 42) take much longer to have any measurable effect on blood sugar. This matters because a quick peak in blood glucose from a high GI carbs stimulates your pancreas to release a large amount of insulin, which in turn causes blood glucose to be transported into glycogen storage. Thus high GI carbs are ideal for quick glycogen replenishment both during and immediately after exercise. However, the large amount of insulin released can result in a reactive 'trough' in blood glucose soon after, making you feel tired, irritable, unable to concentrate and hungry (low blood glucose is a powerful hunger signal for the brain).

Low GI carbs give a slower rise in blood glucose and are therefore not as effective for refuelling either during or immediately after exercise. They don't stimulate the large release of insulin either, and therefore avoid the reactive dip in blood glucose that can follow high GI carbs. So in the long term, you feel more energetic, less irritable, you are able to concentrate and you feel fuller for longer. For this reason, a majority of meals and snacks throughout the day should favour low GI carbs. This promotes a stable blood glucose level, which is the best environment for replenishing muscle glycogen over the longer time-frame.

HOW CAN I TELL IF CARBS ARE HIGH OR LOW GI?

There is a general belief that sugary carbs are fast acting high GI and starchy complex carbs are slow acting and low GI, but this is not the case and the truth is much more complicated. For example, the carbohydrate in apples is all sugar and yet they are low GI. This is because the sugar in apples is mainly in the form of fructose (or 'fruit sugar') which your body takes much longer to digest than glucose. White bread, which contains mainly complex carbohydrates, has a high GI. It happens that the intense processing involved in the production of a modern white loaf makes the starch particles very easy for your body to break down and utilise. Baked potatoes actually have a higher GI than boiled potatoes (it's to do with the cooking process).

The easiest rule to follow is 'unrefined' versus 'refined'. Carbs that are unrefined, such as wholemeal bread, beans, pulses, fruit and vegetables, tend to be slow acting lower GI foods. Whereas refined carbs, such as white bread, breakfast cereals, refined sugar and canned drinks are usually fast acting high GI foods.

One final point about GI: the number only applies to a portion of carbs eaten in isolation. As soon as fats and proteins are combined with the carbs, then the blood glucose spike is slowed significantly. For example, high GI white bread combined with cheese and pickle to make a tasty sandwich, results in a lower GI meal. It is a good plan to eat your carbs as part of a balanced meal or snack that also contains proteins and healthy fats.

PROTEIN SPARING

The body has the ability to make glucose from proteins. The metabolic process is known as gluconeogenesis (literally 'creation of new glucose'). Briefly, muscle protein is broken down to liberate certain amino acids. These can then be converted by the liver into glucose and used for energy.

Breaking down muscle protein in this way is not an ideal situation because it involves cannibalising your own muscles for energy. Instead, your aim should be to consume enough carbs so that your protein is spared for its role in growth and repair. You may hear carbs called 'protein sparing' for this reason.

Glucose can also be made in a very limited way from the glycerol part of triglycerides, the most common form of stored fats in the body, but the quantity produced is not significant.

WHAT IS 'CARBOHYDRATE LOADING'?

Carbohydrate loading is a technique used by marathon runners, long-distance cyclists and triathletes to maximise their muscle glycogen reserves ready for a race. There are many possible carb loading regimens. A popular approach over the week leading up to a race used to be to cut out carbs on the Monday, Tuesday and Wednesday, followed by a high carb intake on the Thursday, Friday and Saturday. The severe glycogen depletion from the first three days led to an over-compensation when carbs are reintroduced, resulting in fuller-than-normal glycogen stores for the start of the race. However, the benefits of this over-compensation are countered by the disrupted training during the depletion phase, making the results of this approach debatable. Most endurance athletes now prefer simply to decrease their training ('taper') and increase their carb intake. A typical carb loading regime is shown here.

	Mon	Tues	Wed	Thurs	Fri	Sat	Sun
Carb intake	Normal	Normal	Normal	High	High	High	Pre-race meal
Training	Normal	Taper	Taper	Taper	Taper/ none	None	Race (e.g. marathon)

Normal carb intake assumes you are already eating around 60% of your calories as carbs anyway. High carb intake in the 2 – 3 days leading up to the event can be as much as 8 – 10g/kg body weight (Sherman, Costill, Fink, & Miller, 1981). For our example people, this equates to Judy eating 496 – 620g carbs and Jack eating 680 – 850g carbs per day. In reality, this is close to doubling their normal intake. It is hard to do this purely from healthy unrefined cereals, fruit and veg. High energy supplements in the form of drinks and gels will probably be necessary.

Another option is to try a one day loading regimen originating in Australia. Training is tapered during the week preceding the event, whilst maintaining your usual carb intake. Then on the day before the race, just one three-minute high intensity training session is performed, followed by full rest and a very high carb intake (10 – 12g/kg body weight, mainly from high GI foods or supplements). The short maximal workout appears to stimulate increased glycogen storage, with levels achieved that are comparable to the six day system (Fairchild & al, 2002) (Bussau & al, 2002).

CARBOHYDRATE SUMMARY

Carbohydrates are essential for energy to exercise, but your body has only limited carb stores (as glycogen) compared to fat. A high carb diet is especially important for endurance events like running a 10k, marathon or triathlon, and there is a wealth of evidence to support this. Carbs should constitute 60% of your normal calorie intake, mainly from unrefined low GI foods, giving steady blood sugar to replenish glycogen over the 24 – 48 hours between intense training sessions. Sufficient carbohydrate has a protein sparing effect, leaving dietary protein available for important growth and repair functions as intended. During and immediately following training, refined high GI carbs are recommended for instant energy and faster initial glycogen replenishment. Prior to an endurance event you may benefit from carb loading to maximise your glycogen stores. Both one week and one day regimens seem to be effective. Experiment during training to find what works best for you.

4

PROTEINS

It has long been recognised that people who exercise need a higher intake of proteins when compared to sedentary individuals. There are three main reasons for this:

- [ ] Exercise increases the stress placed on muscles, tendons, ligaments and bone. Proteins are essential for repair and recovery of these body tissues following exercise.
- [ ] Strength training with weights leads to muscle growth, which requires additional protein.
- [ ] Some of the amino acids from proteins can be metabolised to meet the increased energy demands of exercise. The body does not like to use proteins for energy, preferring instead to use carbs and fats. But if your diet is low in carbs, then proteins become the only option (see Chapter 4).

HOW MUCH PROTEIN SHOULD I EAT?

There has always been much debate on this subject, but the results of various studies and reviews give some useful guidelines which can be summarised as follows:

Activity	Protein intake
Sedentary	0.8g/kg body weight
Endurance (cardiovascular) training	1.2 – 1.4g/kg body weight
Strength/power (weight) training	1.4 – 1.8g/kg body weight

(www.hsph.harvard.edu, 2012) (Phillips S. M., 2012)
(Phillips & van Loon, 2011) (Lemon, 1996)

For example, if Judy, our very active 62kg female from Chapter 2 mainly enjoys endurance training, her daily protein intake should be between:

62 x 1.2 = 74.4g
62 x 1.4 = 86.8g

Let's put these figures into perspective: 1g of protein supplies approximately 4kcal of energy. Thus:

74.4g protein = 297.6kcal
86.6g protein = 346.4kcal

In Chapter 2 we calculated that Judy should eat 2,449kcal total per day. Therefore her protein intake, expressed as a percentage of total energy, equates to:

297.6/2,449 = 12%
346.4/2,449 = 14%

In other words, she will achieve an adequate protein intake simply by following recommended proportions of 12 – 15% of total energy. No other special dietary measures or supplements are needed. This turns out to be the case for a vast majority of people:

A normal, well-balanced diet provides all the protein needed for the demands of exercise.

If Judy decided to change her exercise programme and focus more on resistance training to build strength and power, then she should increase her daily protein intake to between:

62 x 1.4 = 86.8g
62 x 1.8 = 111.6g

The change to strength and power training thus increases her protein requirement to between 14 – 18% of total calories, which may not be covered by normal healthy eating. Additional emphasis should then be placed on eating protein foods, or possibly the use of a supplement to meet the increased demand.

Note that many magazine articles, particularly those associated with bodybuilding, advocate much higher protein intakes, typically between 3 – 4g/kg body weight. However, evidence for the benefits of such high intakes is hard to find, and it is interesting to note that the same magazines that carry these articles also contain dozens of adverts for protein supplements. You can draw your own conclusions.

CAN EXCESSIVE PROTEIN INTAKE BE HARMFUL?

Within reason, a healthy body can cope well with a protein intake greater than you need. Excess proteins are simply converted by the liver into useful glucose, which is then used for energy. The nitrogen part of the protein that is no longer needed is excreted in the urine.

However, there are two possible concerns here. The first is the additional demand placed on your liver and kidneys to deal with the excess protein. Healthy organs will cope with the additional load, but if there is any underlying medical condition they may not. The second is the extra calories: If you constantly over-consume proteins and have no use for the additional energy, then, like all excess calories, they ultimately end up stored as body fat.

WHEN IS THE BEST TIME TO EAT PROTEINS?

Common sense suggests that a regular supply of protein throughout the day will keep circulating blood levels of amino acids high and create the best environment for muscular recovery, growth and repair. Also, there seems to be a limit of around 20 – 25g of protein that your body can use for growth and repair at one time (Phillips & van Loon, 2011). If greater amounts are eaten the excess is simply used as energy or the energy is stored as fat. This implies that protein intake should be spread evenly over meals and snacks throughout the day.

We have already seen that carbs are important for the post-workout recovery snack, and this goes equally for protein. *In fact, evidence suggests that a combination of carbs, protein and fluids gives the best recovery meal.* There is a definite window of opportunity in the 1 – 2 hours immediately after exercise when the body strives to recover. This is the optimum time to supply 20 – 25g of easily digested proteins, making the amino acids available for synthesis of new tissue. A well-balanced meal or snack can easily supply this much protein. Alternatively, a supplement based on whey protein may be a convenient option.

PROTEIN QUALITY

Proteins consist of smaller units called amino acids. Some of these amino acids can be made by the body, but others known as 'essential' amino acids must be obtained from food. Each protein food contains different quantities of these essential amino acids. A high-quality protein food is one that has high levels of essential amino acids that are easily utilised by your body. A high percentage of the protein is retained by your body for tissue growth and repair. A low-quality protein food has one or more of the essential amino acids missing, meaning the body cannot utilise it until the absent amino acids are supplied. This rating of protein quality is called the 'biological value' (BV) and is given a number between 1 and 100. Traditionally, eggs contain such good quality proteins that they are given a BV of 100, and then other protein foods are compared to this. The following table gives examples of high and low BV protein sources.

High BV (70 – 100)	Low BV (below 70)
Eggs	Nuts
Meat	Seeds
Poultry	Pulses
Fish	Wheat
Cheese	Rice
Milk	
Tofu	
Soya milk	

Biological values can be used as a reasonable guide to protein quality. Note that the high BV proteins are mainly from animal sources, whilst lower BV proteins are from non-animal foods. The main exceptions to this rule are soya products (tofu, soya milk, etc.). In practice, it is easy to improve the quality of low BV proteins simply by combining two or more foods together. For example, baked beans on toast combines beans with wheat giving a high BV source of protein. A peanut butter sandwich gives a similar result. Artificially produced whey protein supplements typically have a BV of 105 or higher, which is one of the reasons they are so popular (Chapter 8).

Some authorities, such as the World Health Organization (WHO) and the US Food and Drug Administration (FDA), question the validity of BV when rating proteins. This is because it depends on so many factors such as your age, gender, health, body weight, activity levels and how you cook the food, all of which affect digestibility and ultimate usefulness. They propose instead a 'protein digestibility' score as a more realistic rating, with 1.00 being the highest:

Protein Type	Protein Digestibility Corrected Amino Acid Score (PDCAAS)
Egg	1.00
Milk	1.00
Casein	1.00
Whey protein	1.00
Soy protein	1.00
Beef	0.92
Black beans	0.75
Peanuts	0.52
Wheat gluten	0.25

(Hoffman & Falvo, 2004)

These scores are slightly different to BVs, but follow a similar overall pattern, with egg, milk, soya and meat being superior in amino acid content to beans, nuts and cereals.

FAT CONTENT OF PROTEIN FOODS

Perhaps more importantly than protein quality, the quantity and type of fat associated with that protein source should also be considered. Here is a rough guide:

Fat content of different protein foods		
High in saturated fat	High in unsaturated fat	Low in fat
Eggs	Oily fish	Tofu
Meat (depends on product)	Nuts	Soya milk
Cheese	Seeds	Pulses
Full-fat milk		Wheat
Fish from the chip shop		Rice
		Cottage cheese
		Skimmed milk
		Tuna in brine or spring water
		Lean chicken / turkey breast

Vegetable proteins from wheat, rice and pulses, when eaten in combinations to enhance their BV, can be very useful when aiming for simultaneously high protein and low fat intake. Tofu, soya milk, and low fat dairy, fish, chicken and turkey products are also good choices. The benefits of high quality proteins from eggs, meat and cheese are offset somewhat by their high saturated fat content. Proteins from oily fish, nuts and seeds supply healthy fats in the same package. But note that they still count as high fat foods and calories from healthy fats can still make you fat, so avoid excessive consumption.

PROTEIN SUMMARY

For endurance cardiovascular training, eat 1.2 – 1.4g/kg body weight each day. For strength training, eat 1.4 – 1.8g/kg body weight per day. This typically equates to between 12 – 20% of total daily calories.

Digestibility and assimilation at one serving is limited to about 20 – 25g. Therefore, protein intake should be divided evenly over meals and snacks throughout the day. Protein quality is as important as quantity; you can use BV or protein digestibility scores as a guide. Also, consider quantity and type of fats associated with that protein source.

Combinations of vegetable proteins are a useful way to provide high quality proteins whilst minimising fat intake. In the immediate post-workout period is particularly important to eat 20 – 25g of easily digested proteins, preferably in combination with high GI carbs to aid absorption.

5

FATS

Nutrition for exercise tends to focus primarily on carbs and proteins for reasons we have already discussed, yet there are many important roles played by fats in terms of general health, fuelling long exercise sessions, and promoting ideal hormonal conditions for recovery after training. Fats have the following important functions:

- ☐ They are integral to cell membranes and are important for growth and repair of body tissues.
- ☐ They are a major constituent of brain tissue and insulation of nerves.
- ☐ They contain the 'fat soluble' vitamins A, D, E and K.
- ☐ Omega 3 and Omega 6 essential fatty acids (EFAs) are vital for a wide range of functions.
- ☐ Body fat offers insulation and protection, and it is a store of energy that we can call on during long training sessions.
- ☐ Body fat is particularly important in women for production and regulation of hormones.

VERY LOW FAT DIETS

The list of roles for fat is quite extensive, so it is not surprising that a very low fat diet can cause health problems such as poor skin and hair condition, reduced vitamin status and hormonal deficiencies. Fats are also important for taste, texture and flavour of foods. A diet entirely devoid of fats is extremely bland and unpalatable. So fats are vital, but they have to be healthy fats and they have to be eaten in the right quantity.

HOW MUCH FAT SHOULD I EAT?

Basic healthy eating guidelines advise us to consume no more than 30 – 35% of total calories from fats (www.bda.uk.com, 2013), (www.nhs.uk, 2013) For many people who train at a moderate level this is about right, leaving 55 – 60% to come from carbs and 10 – 15% to come from proteins. However, for a high-performance diet for exercise, both carb and protein intakes need to be higher and hence the fat calories must be reduced accordingly. A useful guideline is to aim for 20 – 25% of total calories from fat.

At first sight 20 – 25% of total calories may seem easily achievable. But consider that fat intake for the population in general is closer to 40% of calories, and that fat is important for food taste and texture, and for general eating pleasure. Also consider that fat is very calorie dense (9kcal per g) when compared to carbs or proteins (4kcal per g). So, in reality, 25% of calories from fat will not equate to 25% of the bulk of your food you see on your plate; it is actually much less. Keeping your fat intake to just 20 – 25% takes conscious effort and careful food choices.

WHAT TYPES OF FAT SHOULD I EAT?

When choosing types of fat, eating for exercise follows the same rules as healthy eating. Fats that are mainly liquid at room temperature are classified as 'unsaturated' and examples include sunflower oil, olive oil, nuts, seeds and oily fish like mackerel or salmon. Unsaturated fats are therefore mainly vegetable oils and fish oils. Unsaturated fats are generally classified as healthy because they have a beneficial effect on your blood lipoprotein ('cholesterol') levels and they also contain good levels of omega 3 and omega 6 EFAs. Unsaturated fats can be further subdivided into 'monounsaturated' and 'polyunsaturated'.

Fats that are mainly solid at room temperature are classified as 'saturated' and examples include butter, lard, cheese, suet, and fat on meat such as bacon or steak. Saturated fats are usually animal fats, although palm oil and coconut oil are exceptions to this rule. Pizza and cheese are the biggest food sources of saturated fat in the diet, and other dairy and meat products are also major contributors (www.hsph.harvard.edu, 2012). Saturated fats are generally classified as unhealthy because they have a harmful effect on your blood lipoprotein levels.

Processing of fats using hydrogenation is a specific concern. The hydrogenation process results in some harmful 'trans-fats' being present in the food. These have a particularly harmful effect on your blood lipoprotein levels and other health consequences. You are well advised to eliminate trans-fats from your diet. Food products that may contain trans-fats include: ready meals, chips, crisps, cakes and biscuits. A good rule is to be cautious with any highly processed products.

The following table summarises the different types of fat:

Saturated	Mono/polyunsaturated	Products that may also contain 'trans-fats'
Butter	Olive oil	Ready meals
Lard	Rapeseed oil	Chips
Cheese	Nuts	Crisps
Cream	Seeds	Cakes
Meat fat	Avocados	Biscuits
Fat in cakes & biscuits	Vegetable oils	Snack bars
Palm oil	Oily fish	Doughnuts
Coconut oil		Chocolate
		Spreads (margarines)

ESSENTIAL FATTY ACIDS

Omega 3 and 6 EFAs are specific types of fat found predominantly in unsaturated oils from fish, seeds and nuts. An adequate intake of omega 3 EFAs reduces blood clotting, having the effect of 'thinning the blood' and helping to lower blood pressure. This in turn reduces your chances of getting a blocked artery or suffering from a heart attack. There are also anti-inflammatory effects which can be beneficial to your joints, and it is possible that improved circulation and blood flow can improve cardiovascular exercise performance. Omega 6 EFAs are vital for healthy structure and functioning of cell membranes and particularly important for healthy skin.

A typical diet in today's developed countries is plentiful in omega 6 because of widespread use of vegetable oils. In contrast, omega 3 consumption is more limited and authorities agree that we would benefit from a higher intake. The most effective way to do this is to include 2 – 3 portions of oily fish like mackerel or salmon in the diet each week. If you don't like the taste of oily fish, or if you are vegetarian, then seeds and nuts also contain significant quantities of omega 3. Many products like spreads, yoghurts, bread and eggs now have omega 3 added as part of the production process. Note that large doses of omega 3 EFAs can have a significant effect on blood clotting times. Anyone already taking blood thinning medication should consult their doctor before using fish oil supplements.

FATS SUMMARY

Dietary fats are essential to health. Frequent exercisers should aim to eat 20 – 25% of their calories from fats, which is lower than an average intake and implies careful food choices and preparation methods to limit fat content. For health reasons, the majority of fats should come from unsaturated fat sources such as nuts, seeds, oily fish and vegetable oils. Oily fish are particularly important because they are a good source of omega 3 EFA. When eating animal fats choose better quality products rather than processed. Eliminate from your diet as far as possible any products that contain trans-fats.

6

VITAMINS, MINERALS AND PHYTOCHEMICALS

It is generally recognised that the need for vitamins, minerals (micronutrients) and phytochemicals increases with an intense exercise programme. This is particularly true of specific micronutrients involved in energy production, in maintaining the immune system, or in the recovery process. However, this does not necessarily imply that special dietary measures need to be taken to ensure an adequate supply – nor does it mean resorting to a supplement. This is because the active individual will take in more total food than their inactive counterpart. So long as the quality of the extra food remains high and conforms to the healthy eating plate, then micronutrient intake is automatically increased.

Active people can meet their micronutrient requirements simply by eating a healthy diet.

If you suspect you may have a specific deficiency then consult a dietician for professional advice. Indiscriminate supplementation is not recommended and can do more harm than good. Having said this, there are certain circumstances where care should be taken and where supplementation may be appropriate. Here are some considerations.

RESTRICTING FOOD INTAKE TO LOSE WEIGHT

Sometimes you may need to restrict food intake to lose weight whilst trying to maintain a training schedule. Calorie restriction should never be so severe that you starve your body (see Chapter 2), but even within the guidelines for safe weight loss and maintaining a balanced diet, it is inevitable that your vitamin and mineral status will decline. In such circumstances the use of a multivitamin and mineral supplement may be beneficial.

VITAMIN D

Vitamin D is essential for bone health. This is because it acts as a hormone allowing the bones to absorb and fix calcium within their structure to maintain bone strength and density. Deficiency of vitamin D causes softening of the bones in children (rickets) and bone weakening conditions such as osteomalacia and osteoporosis in adults.

Vitamin D is fat-soluble and therefore comes in foods such as butter, margarines (where extra vitamin D is added), oily fish, eggs and dairy products. Vitamin D can also be made by the skin when exposed to sunlight. This means that your vitamin D intake could be compromised if you:

- ☐ Are on a very low fat diet
- ☐ Don't get much exposure to sunlight (i.e. because you are indoors a lot, you live in a cold country with restricted daylight, you wear clothing that covers your body or you habitually use sunscreen)

If you think you are at risk of vitamin D deficiency then seek medical advice and have your status properly tested (Powers S, 2011).

CALCIUM

You probably already know that calcium is a major mineral constituent of bones and teeth. It is especially important for adolescents because of skeletal growth, and for post-menopausal women because of the increased risk of osteoporosis. If you follow the healthy eating food plate and consume at least three portions of dairy products daily, then this will supply adequate calcium. Note that low fat dairy products have similar calcium content to the full fat versions. If you cannot, or do not want to, consume dairy foods then other options include: green leafy vegetables, such as broccoli and cabbage, soya beans and tofu (soya bean curd), soya drinks with added calcium, nuts, bread and anything made with fortified flour (which has calcium added to it) and fish where you eat the bones, such as sardines (www.nhs.uk, 2012).

IRON

The mineral iron is very commonly deficient in the diet, particularly if you are restricting calories, if you are vegetarian or vegan, or if you simply avoid eating red meat. Iron is used by the body to form haemoglobin which is a part of red blood cells and used to carry oxygen around the body. Anyone deficient in iron has reduced oxygen transport to their muscles, which severely limits aerobic energy production, making them feel tired very quickly. This condition of iron deficiency leading to chronic tiredness is known as anaemia. Women are at a higher risk of anaemia than men because of regular menstrual blood loss, and because of a generally lower dietary intake in the first place. Iron is the only micronutrient where the guideline daily amount for women is higher than for men.

Regular supplementation with iron is not recommended because it can quickly become toxic. Instead, the best strategy to avoid anaemia is to eat iron-rich foods. Liver, kidney and red meat generally are the best sources of easily absorbed iron. Significant quantities are also found in breakfast cereals fortified with iron, eggs, legumes and green leafy vegetables, but they are poorly absorbed, meaning that a lot of their iron content simply passes through the gut. Vitamin C from fruit and veg will aid absorption levels to some extent.

OXYGEN FREE RADICALS AND ANTIOXIDANTS

Antioxidants are substances found in food that help to prevent cellular damage from oxygen free radicals. Free radicals are inevitable by-products of respiration and oxygen use in the body. They are very unstable molecules and can damage cells unless they are neutralised, or 'quenched', by antioxidants. The most effective antioxidants from food are vitamin A (meat, eggs, whole milk, butter), beta carotene (brightly coloured fruit and veg), vitamin C (fresh fruit and veg), vitamin E (wheat germ, fruit, nuts, cereals) and selenium (brazil nuts, fish, eggs, sunflower seeds). A number of phytochemicals also function as antioxidants.

PHYTOCHEMICALS

Phytochemicals are substances found in plants that can have a beneficial effect on our health ('phyto' is from the Greek indicating 'plant'). You may have heard results of research saying that red wine, grapes, berries, garlic, onions, tea, tomatoes and broccoli are all good for us. This advice is usually based on phytochemicals they contain, such as carotenoids and flavonoids. Although phytochemicals are not counted as essential nutrients, many of them appear to have a significant protective effect against the development of heart disease and cancer. This is possibly why there is a strong link between eating lots of plant foods and a lowered risk of suffering from these health problems.

Exercise increases respiration rates and therefore increases the body's production of oxygen free radicals, so a higher intake of antioxidant phytochemicals should help to quench these additional free radicals. But, as with vitamins and minerals, evidence suggests that the body naturally increases its defences against increased oxidative stress, and that the additional calorie intake from being active will easily meet the extra demand, assuming it is balanced correctly to contain lots of fruit and veg. Indeed, recent research points to free radicals being important as part of the response to exercise that leads to adaptations.

VITAMINS, MINERALS AND PHYTOCHEMICALS SUMMARY

The need for vitamins, minerals and phytochemicals increases with an intense exercise programme. However, active individuals will eat more food than their sedentary counterparts. So long as the quality of the extra food remains high and conforms to the healthy eating plate, then micronutrient intake is automatically increased. If you are restricting food intake to lose weight then a multivitamin and mineral supplement may be useful to ensure adequate intake (see Chapter 8). Deficiencies of vitamin D, calcium and iron are possible under certain circumstances, but indiscriminate supplementation is not recommended. Consult a dietician for professional advice.

7

HYDRATION

Adequate hydration is vital to physical performance. If you allow yourself to become mildly dehydrated then exercise capacity starts to fall: the heart has to work harder to circulate blood and oxygen to your muscles, cellular energy production is slowed, and you are less able to cool your body. If you are mildly dehydrated then the natural response is to feel thirsty and this will prompt you to have a drink. It takes a while, though, for the fluid to be absorbed from the gut and reach your cells to restore you to a fully hydrated state and your performance will suffer during this time. Hence you should avoid dehydration in the first place by drinking adequately before, during and after exercise.

If you are unable to drink and become severely dehydrated then you will experience symptoms such as headache, dry mouth, nausea, dizziness and vomiting. In the extreme, dehydration can be fatal. But this is unlikely under normal circumstances.

Your body loses fluid each day just through natural processes and functions. Most fluid is lost as:

- ☐ sweat
- ☐ urine
- ☐ faeces
- ☐ water vapour in breath

There may be other less significant fluid losses from tears, bleeding, mucus, etc. On a typical sedentary day these daily losses total about 2 – 2.5 litres, so it follows that you need to replace this quantity of fluid to remain hydrated. However, note that food itself contains water, so even if you drank nothing in a day you would still obtain about one litre of fluid just from eating. Hence the general guideline for sedentary people is to drink about 1 – 1.5 litres (6 – 8 glasses) of plain water each day, enough to prevent thirst. If you don't like the idea of drinking just plain water, remember that most drinks consist mainly of water and, contrary to received wisdom, will rehydrate to some extent. This includes tea, coffee, cans of cola, beer, milk and fruit juice. They may not be ideal, because of their caffeine, sugar and alcohol content, but they do all contribute to fluid intake and can keep you hydrated.

HOW CAN I TELL IF I AM FULLY HYDRATED?

Your body will detect mild dehydration and this will make you feel thirsty, which will prompt you to have a drink and rehydrate. If you are losing larger volumes of fluid as sweat because of exercise or humidity, you will feel thirstier and drink more – a simple feedback loop that has served humans well for thousands of years. Mild dehydration will also lead to darker coloured urine and reduced urine volume. Clear or pale 'straw coloured' urine is a reliable indicator of hydration. So if you don't feel thirsty and urine colour is clear or pale yellow, you can be confident you are fully hydrated (note: if your urine is bright yellow after taking a vitamin supplement, don't worry, it's a side effect of vitamin B2, not dehydration).

Drinking more water than you need has no additional benefits. You will simply excrete it as urine a while later and it does no harm. During exercise, drinking too much can make you feel bloated and cause abdominal discomfort, so it is definitely not recommended. Be aware that there are extreme circumstances usually associated with illness or endurance races, where too much water can dilute the sodium in the blood (see 'Do I need extra salt?').

FLUID REQUIREMENTS AND EXERCISE

Frequent exercise, larger body size or hot and humid weather – all of these factors can increase your fluid needs considerably above the 1 – 1.5 litres baseline for sedentary people.

If you are active, a reasonable estimate of fluid requirements can be made based around your daily energy expenditure:

For every 1,000kcal of energy you expend, drink a minimum of 1 litre of fluids, mostly as plain water.

Take your daily energy expenditure calculated in Chapter 2, then use the table that follows as an easy reference.

Daily energy expenditure (kcal)	Recommended fluid intake (litres)
2,500	2.5
3,000	3
3,500	3.5
4,000	4
4,500	4.5

CAN SPORTS DRINKS HELP ME TO REHYDRATE?

Sports drinks labelled as *hypotonic* (2 – 4g sugar/100ml) or *isotonic* (4 – 8g sugar/100ml) may be able to hydrate you a little faster than plain water. This is because they contain small amounts of sugars and salts (*electrolytes*) that help absorption of the water from the stomach into your blood and cells. The sugar content also supplies some energy to help fuel your training. However, it is debatable whether the small advantage they give is significant for most exercise sessions unless they last longer than one hour.

Some sports drinks come under the heading of energy drinks (more than 8g sugar/100ml) because of their high sugar content. Although they do supply energy, the greater sugar content slows absorption of fluid from your stomach and their ability to rehydrate quickly is reduced. Most energy drinks also contain significant amounts of caffeine. The pros and cons of this are discussed more fully in the next chapter.

Your choice of sports drink will therefore depend upon your priority: fast rehydration or energy? The following table summarises the benefits of each class of sports drink compared to plain water.

Poor *   Good **   Very good ***

Drink	Sugar content (per 100ml)	Fast rehydration	Energy
Water	None	**	None
Hypotonic drink	2 – 4g	***	*
Isotonic drink	4 – 8g	***	**
Energy drink	More than 8g	*	***

As you can see, the best compromise between fast rehydration and energy content is an isotonic drink. You will find that the most common commercial brands are isotonic for this reason.

DO I NEED EXTRA SALT?

Salt is essential to hydration. This is because the sodium ions found in salt (sodium chloride) are important for transport of fluid across cell membranes. However, most people obtain more than enough salt from their normal diet. In fact, most of us consume nearly double the recommended 6g a day (www.nhs.uk, 2012). So the general answer to the question is no, you don't need any extra salt.

If you exercise in a hot climate and lose a lot of sweat over an extended period of several hours, then adding extra salt to a sports drink becomes a sensible idea. Sweat contains a lot of salt, particularly if you are a 'salty sweater', so if you sweat profusely enough for long enough, then low sodium levels in the blood become a real possibility, causing a serious condition called hyponatraemia. This affects the viscosity of the blood which, in turn, affects circulation. Symptoms of hyponatraemia include dizziness and mental confusion. Severe cases can result in circulatory failure and death. Consult a dietician if you have any concerns.

Most commercial brands of sports drink will already contain some salt (check the label). If you are making your own, then about ⅓ of a teaspoon (1- 1.5g) per litre of drink is a useful guideline.

MAKING YOUR OWN SPORTS DRINK

You can mix your own sports drink at home quite easily and save a lot of money. You need a measuring jug and some orange squash or fruit juice. For an isotonic drink the measures are:

1. 1 litre of water
2. Orange squash or fruit juice, enough to contain 60g sugar (check the nutrition label and measure out the right amount)
3. ⅓ of a teaspoon of salt (optional)

HYDRATION BEFORE, DURING AND AFTER EXERCISE

Before starting exercise make sure you are fully hydrated. In practice, this means you need to drink about 500ml of water in the two hours preceding training. If you start a training session already dehydrated it is too late for any fluid intake to have much beneficial effect, even if you drink immediately.

During exercise drink small amounts regularly. It is hard to quantify exactly how much you should drink because this depends so much on your body size, the type of training, how hot it is, how much you sweat, and so on. Find what works best for you. For exercise sessions lasting up to one hour in duration, plain water is recommended. For sessions longer than one hour you will benefit from using an isotonic sports drink containing some carbohydrates and electrolytes. For ultra-distance events the need for carbohydrate for energy may exceed the need for fluid replacement, in which case an energy drink (probably containing caffeine as well) is the preferred choice.

After exercise you should aim to replace all fluids lost during the session. The easiest way to estimate fluid loss is to weigh yourself accurately before and after training. Interestingly, 1kg of weight lost equates almost exactly to one litre of fluid loss. For example if Judy, our 62kg person from Chapter 2, weighs herself after running a 10k and finds she now weighs 60.5kg, this indicates a loss of 1.5 litres of fluid. Over the next 1-2 hours she should aim to drink this much to regain full hydration.

SHOULD I DRINK ALCOHOL?

There is absolutely no need for humans to drink alcohol and this is especially true for anyone involved in exercise. Alcohol serves no nutritional purpose, it is toxic and if you drink enough it can kill you. Alcoholic drinks are also high in calories and contribute significantly to gaining body fat. In the short term, alcohol is a diuretic and will dehydrate the body leading to reduced performance. Compare the symptoms of dehydration (headache, nausea, dry mouth, etc.) to those of a hangover and you find they are very similar. So if you are at all interested in exercise and performance then you will avoid alcohol altogether.

Having said all this, alcohol in moderation can actually have some positive health benefits. It can help people to cope with stress, relax, unwind and be more sociable, there is a small but noticeable blood thinning effect, and certain drinks like red wine, beer and stout contain vitamins, minerals and antioxidants. So if a daily glass of wine or beer is important to you it isn't essential to give it up. Instead, the key phrase here is *in moderation*.

The easiest way to check that you are keeping to a moderate intake is to stay within your 'lower risk guidelines' per day.

Women should not exceed 2 – 3 units per day. This is roughly equivalent to a 175mm glass of wine.
Men should not exceed 3 – 4 units per day. This is roughly equivalent to a strong pint of beer, lager or cider (www.nhs.uk, 2012).

HYDRATION SUMMARY

Drink about 500ml of water within the two hours preceding training to make sure you are fully hydrated. During exercise drink small amounts regularly. For exercise sessions lasting up to one hour, plain water is recommended. For sessions longer than one hour you will benefit from using an isotonic sports drink containing some carbohydrates and electrolytes. For ultra-distance events an energy drink containing carbs and caffeine is the preferred choice. Find out what strategy works best for you. After exercise you should aim to replace all fluids lost during the session. You can weigh yourself before and after training bearing in mind that 1kg of weight lost equates almost exactly to one litre of water. Moderate your alcohol intake or eliminate it completely; it leads to dehydration which can reduce your training performance.

8

SUPPLEMENTS

There is a huge range of supplements available to the exercise enthusiast. The challenge is to decide which ones actually offer some benefit and which are just based on specious 'research' and clever marketing. The supplements discussed here are the most common ones encountered at the gym or health food shop, with good evidence to show that they are beneficial in the right circumstances. But do remember that a supplement is just that – an addition to your usual diet. No supplement can fully overcome the deficiencies of a diet that is poor in the first place.

PROTEIN

Supplements commonly available are based on four different protein sources: whey, casein, soya and egg. They are all excellent sources of complete protein with all of the amino acids necessary for tissue repair and growth. Each protein source has its own specific characteristics:

Protein source	Characteristics
Whey (from milk)	Easy to digest, fast absorption, high BV, ideal for immediately after training
Casein (from milk)	Slow to digest and absorb. Ideal for sustaining blood amino acid levels over a long period (e.g. at bedtime).
Soya (from soya beans)	Suitable for vegetarians, more concentrated amino acids than soya milk or tofu. Easy to digest, fast absorption, high BV, high concentrations of 'branched chain' amino acids essential for muscle growth.
Egg (from whole egg)	'Whole food' protein source, high BV. Now largely superseded by whey and soya products.

By far, the most common of the four are supplements based on whey protein. This is because of their high BV and their fast absorption, making 20 – 25g ideal as part of a recovery meal. Soy isolate also makes a quickly absorbed protein following a workout (Tang, Moore, Kujbida, Tarnopolsky, & Phillips, 2009). Casein-based products are more suited to maintaining blood amino acid levels over several hours making it a good bedtime supplement.

CARBOHYDRATE (ENERGY GELS AND DRINKS)

Energy gels and drinks are of particular interest to the endurance athlete. They contain quickly digested carbs (e.g. glucose) for use during a training session and for speedy replenishment of muscle glycogen afterwards. Energy drinks will also supply significant fluids too, but remember that the high carb content can slow down rehydration compared to water or isotonic drinks. Many commercial energy drinks contain a glucose polymer called *maltodextrin*. This is an artificial product manufactured from wheat or corn starch and consists of molecules somewhere between a sugar and a starch in size. Using a glucose polymer allows the energy drink to supply the equivalent carbs of a glucose drink but contained in fewer particles. This means it can supply the same energy but not slow the rehydration rate.

PROTEIN AND CARBOHYDRATE COMBINATION

Supplements that combine proteins and carbs are usually referred to as 'liquid meals' or 'mass builders' depending upon context. Typically they will provide 20 – 25g of protein and 60 – 80g carbs in an easily digestible liquid form. Products will often also contain a range of vitamins and minerals. These supplements can be a very convenient way to obtain all the major nutrients needed for recovery after training. But do keep in mind that normal food, such as a large bowl of cereal with semi-skimmed milk, will give essentially the same result.

CREATINE

Creatine supplementation aims to increase the stores of high-energy phosphocreatine in the muscles. This can lead to improved energy to train for explosive activities like sprinting, jumping, throwing or weight lifting (Chapter 2). There may also be resultant gains in strength and muscle mass, although evidence suggests that much of the increased body weight experienced on creatine supplementation is due to fluid retention (Powers & al, 2003). This may be a concern if you compete in a weight category sport. Creatine is legal to use and it is now so commonplace that you can buy it at the supermarket. The usual supplement form is *creatine monohydrate* powder, although other forms are available. Creatine supplements have been in widespread use since the early 1990s and do not appear to be harmful to health.

CAFFEINE

Caffeine affects our central nervous system and has many proven performance benefits, particularly in terms of mental concentration, fat utilisation and long-term endurance. The amount required to have any significant effect on performance is about 3 – 6mg/kg body weight (Ganio, Klau, Casa, Armstrong, & Maresh, 2009). So for Judy from Chapter 2, this equates to 186 – 372mg, which is equivalent to 2 – 4 strong coffees, 2 – 4 cans of energy drink, or 4 – 8 cans of cola. On the downside, caffeine is a known diuretic. In other words, it stimulates increased urine production, which may lead to dehydration.

Individual response to caffeine varies widely with some people feeling little effect, whilst others experience sleep disorders and anxiety. Also, regular coffee or cola drinkers rapidly build up a tolerance to caffeine making both the stimulant effect and the dehydration less significant. If you want to make use of caffeine as a performance enhancing supplement, then do so in a targeted way, using the correct amount only when you need it. Indiscriminate use will build up your tolerance and reduce potential effectiveness.

VITAMINS AND MINERALS

In Chapter 6 we covered the general increased need for vitamins and minerals for the active compared to the sedentary individual. We also stated that a well-balanced diet that supplies all the necessary calories will also supply enough of the micronutrients too. Despite this, many people still believe in taking vitamin and mineral supplements just to make sure their intake is sufficient. This is sensible when:

☐ work, travel and family commitments mean that your diet is less than ideal
☐ you are restricting your food intake to lose weight
☐ you don't eat certain food groups due to allergy

If you do decide to take a supplement, then a broad-range multivitamin and mineral is the best choice. Check on the product label that:

☐ A full range of vitamins and minerals are included
☐ Quantities are somewhere close to 100% of the guideline daily amount (GDA) for each nutrient. In particular, mega doses of *minerals* should be avoided because any excess can quickly become toxic

Avoid excessive supplementation of just one vitamin or mineral (unless it's following your doctor's advice). Micronutrients are 'team players' – they work best in combination. If you mega-dose just one, then this can negatively affect the absorption or action of another. Also be aware that many other foods are fortified with vitamins and minerals, so you may be taking in more than you think. These include white flour and breakfast cereals (B vitamins, calcium and iron), soya flour and milk (calcium), margarines/spreads (vitamins A, D and E) and so on.

BUFFERING AGENTS

Sports that use the anaerobic energy systems for several minutes, such as 800m or 1500m running, or 2000m rowing, will accumulate high levels of lactate/H^+ ions in the blood. In principle, if you can take a supplement that makes your blood more alkaline, then this will 'buffer' the rise in acidity, enabling you to train at high intensity for longer before the pain becomes unbearable and the muscles stop working. Sodium bicarbonate is a commonly available alkaline powder that can be used in this way (similar to taking bicarbonate tablets to neutralise stomach acidity).

Both anecdotal and research evidence suggests that this strategy can work. However, a major side effect from taking sodium bicarbonate is an upset stomach. So it is wise to experiment during training to evaluate the benefits versus the side effects for you as an individual.

9

SUMMARY GUIDELINES FOR WEIGHT TRAINING

If your main interest is weight training for strength, power or muscle gain, then the following are the most important nutrition guidelines for you. Note that good nutrition is only one factor necessary for developing muscle strength and size. Also important are effective training, adequate recovery, body type and genetics. You can follow the best diet but still not make the same gains as the next person simply because they have more favourable genetics.

ENERGY

Calorie intake should be high enough to support training and maintenance of lean muscle. Use the Schofield equation and PAF to estimate your individual needs then refine this based on your experience and progress.

If you want to gain lean muscle rather than just maintain what you have, then you will need to increase your calorie intake significantly more than your maintenance level. Increasing your energy intake by 20% is recommended (Bean, 2003). Judy and Jack from Chapter 2 required 2,449kcal and 3,753kcal respectively for maintenance purposes. If they wished to gain lean muscle, then they would need:

Judy: 2,449 + 20%   Jack: 3,753 + 20%
        = 2,449 + 490   = 3,753 + 750
        = 2,939kcal   = 4,503 kcal

These additional calories should maintain the normal balance between fats, carbs and proteins. But be warned: simply eating lots of extra calories will lead to fat gain. The extra calories must be combined with intense resistance training for gains in lean weight.

CARBOHYDRATE

Weight training is almost exclusively anaerobic, thus relying on stores of glycogen as the primary fuel for your workout. Carb intake should therefore be maintained at 60% of total calories to give full glycogen replenishment between training sessions. Meals and snacks should be based mainly on unrefined low GI carbs to give the steady blood glucose level most effective for glycogen storage. An exception to the low GI rule is the post-training meal/snack where high GI carbs are recommended within the first hour to stimulate rapid initial glycogen storage.

PROTEIN

A protein intake of 1.4 – 1.8g/kg of your body weight is sufficient to provide all the amino acids you need for muscle maintenance, repair and growth. Utilisation of protein in the body at any one time is limited to about 20 – 25g; therefore your total protein intake should be spread evenly over 4 – 6 meals/snacks throughout the day. If you find it hard to consume this amount of protein then a supplement may be a convenient way to make up any shortfall. The post-training meal is a particularly important time to eat some easily digested proteins.

PRE-TRAINING

Eat a meal/snack high in carbs about 2 – 3 hours before your workout to give you energy to train. Most authorities advocate a low GI carb to maintain a steady blood sugar during your session. A high GI carb carries the risk of a rebound low blood sugar just when you are about to exercise. A common practice is to have a whey protein supplement just before training, the idea being to prevent muscle breakdown during the session. Most research suggests that post-training is the critical time for protein.

POST-TRAINING

Within the first hour following a weight training session you should consume a meal/snack that is high in both proteins and carbs; 20 – 25g of high-quality proteins and 60 – 80g of high GI carbs gives a useful guideline. Examples of foods that will supply this include:

☐ A bowl of pasta (100g dry weight) with some tuna (small 60g tin)
☐ A bowl of rice (100g dry weight) with some chicken (100g)
☐ Two medium baked potatoes with cottage cheese (150g)

If you are unable to cook food immediately after training, then you will need to prepare it in advance. Alternatively, a supplement can be more convenient. Many health clubs will serve these in their café or juice bar. Commercial products like these will often contain a range of vitamins and minerals too.

FAT

Fats are not used as a fuel for weight training. However, fats are essential for the recovery process. They are also important for maintaining levels of anabolic (muscle building) hormones. An intake of 20 – 25% of your total calories from healthy fats is a realistic target.

VITAMINS, MINERALS AND PHYTONUTRIENTS

The general increase in calories for training will provide all the micronutrients you need, provided that the balance of food groups still follows the healthy eating plate.

HYDRATION

Begin your workout fully hydrated by drinking 500ml of water in the two hours preceding training. The intermittent nature of weight training, with sets followed by long rest periods, doesn't lead to much fluid loss from sweating and so makes hydration during a workout less important. Sipping a drink occasionally to cleanse the palate is fine.

SUPPLEMENTS

The main supplements that can help with weight training for strength, power or muscle gain are: whey, soya and casein protein powders, protein and carb 'mass builders', and creatine monohydrate (see Chapter 8).

10

SUMMARY GUIDELINES FOR CARDIOVASCULAR TRAINING

If your main interest is cardiovascular training, such as running, cycling, swimming or triathlon, then the following are the most important nutrition guidelines for you.

ENERGY

This should be high enough to support training and maintenance of lean muscle. Use the Schofield equation and PAF to estimate your individual needs then refine this based on your experience and progress. If you use high volumes of training regularly, then it is worthwhile measuring exactly how many calories you need.

CARBOHYDRATE

Endurance training mainly utilises the aerobic energy system, with some contribution from the anaerobic systems at high intensity. Thus your training sessions rely on a mix of fat and glycogen as the primary fuels, but as discussed in Chapters 2 and 3, it is your glycogen stores that are the limiting factor, not your fat stores. Carb intake should therefore be maintained at 60% of total calories to give full glycogen replenishment between training sessions. Meals and snacks should be based mainly on unrefined low GI carbs to give the steady blood glucose level most effective for glycogen storage. An exception to the low GI rule is the post-training meal/snack where high GI carbs are recommended within the first hour to stimulate rapid initial glycogen storage.

If you regularly complete training sessions or events that last longer than 90 minutes, then carb intake during training is important. This is most convenient in the form of energy drinks or gels. Aim to take in 60g of carbs for every hour of exercise (Coggan & Coyle, 1991). Carbohydrate loading can be useful prior to an event. See Chapter 3 for guidelines about one week or one day regimes.

PROTEIN

A protein intake of 1.2 – 1.4g/kg of your body weight is sufficient to provide all the amino acids you need for muscle maintenance and repair. Utilisation of protein in the body at any one time is limited to about 20 – 25g; therefore your total protein intake should be spread evenly over 4 – 6 meals/snacks throughout the day. Your normal food intake, provided it is well balanced, will easily provide this amount of protein. The post-training meal is a particularly important time to eat some easily digested proteins.

PRE-TRAINING

Eat a meal/snack high in carbs about 2 – 3 hours before your workout to give you energy to train. For long sessions 2.5g carbs/kg body weight is recommended. Most authorities advocate a low GI carb to maintain a steady blood sugar during your session. A high GI carb carries the risk of a rebound low blood sugar just when you are about to exercise.

POST-TRAINING

Within the first hour following a weight training session you should consume a meal/snack that contains 20 - 25g of high-quality proteins to facilitate muscle repair. If your goal is to build muscle mass, then the protein should be accompanied with about 60 - 80g of high GI carbs to stimulate insulin release for rapid glycogen replenishment and for transport of proteins from the blood into the cells.

FAT

Fats are used as a fuel for cardiovascular training, particularly in ultra-distance events. But this does not mean you need a high intake. Consuming 20 – 25% of your total calories from healthy fats is a realistic target. Fats are also essential for the recovery process and for maintaining levels of anabolic (muscle building) hormones.

VITAMINS, MINERALS AND PHYTONUTRIENTS

The general increase in calories for training will provide all the micronutrients you need, provided that the balance of food groups still follows the healthy eating plate.

HYDRATION

Begin your workout fully hydrated by drinking 500ml of water in the two hours preceding training. During exercise drink small amounts regularly. For exercise sessions lasting up to one hour in duration, plain water is recommended. For longer sessions you will benefit from using an isotonic sports drink or an energy drink. After training you should aim to replace all fluids lost during the session. Weighing yourself accurately before and after training can determine how much water you have lost (1kg weight loss = almost exactly to 1 litre of water loss).

SUPPLEMENTS

The main supplements that can help with cardiovascular training are: protein and carb 'mass builders' for a recovery snack, energy drinks and gels, caffeine, and buffering agents (if you compete in events which build up high levels of lactic acid).

BIBLIOGRAPHY

www.choosemyplate.gov. (2012). Retrieved November 24, 2012, from http://www.choosemyplate.gov/food-groups
ymcaed.org.uk/fg

www.dh.gov.uk. (2012). Retrieved November 24, 2012, from http://www.dh.gov.uk/health/2012/06/about-the-eatwell-plate
ymcaed.org.uk/abe

www.hsph.harvard.edu. (2012). Retrieved November 24, 2012, from http://www.hsph.harvard.edu/nutritionsource/what-should-you-eat/pyramid-full-story/index.html
ymcaed.org.uk/pyr

www.hsph.harvard.edu. (2012). Retrieved November 24, 2012, from http://www.hsph.harvard.edu/nutritionsource/what-should-you-eat/top-food-sources-of-saturated-fat-in-the-us/index.html
ymcaed.org.uk/sat

www.hsph.harvard.edu. (2012). Retrieved December 23, 2012, from Harvard School of Public Health: http://www.hsph.harvard.edu/nutritionsource/protein-full-story
ymcaed.org.uk/pfs

www.nhs.uk. (2012). Retrieved November 25, 2012, from
http://www.nhs.uk/Change4Life/Pages/change-for-life.aspx
ymcaed.org.uk/c4l

www.nhs.uk. (2012). Retrieved November 24, 2012, from
http://www.nhs.uk/Conditions/vitamins-minerals/Pages/Calcium.aspx
ymcaed.org.uk/cal

www.nhs.uk. (2012). Retrieved December 1, 2012, from
http://www.nhs.uk/Livewell/Goodfood/Pages/salt.aspx
ymcaed.org.uk/sal

Bean, A. (2003). The Complete Guide to Sports Nutrition, 4th edition.
London: A & C Black Publishers Ltd.

Bussau, V., Fairchild, T. J., Rao, A., Steele, P., & Fournier, P. A. (2002).
Carbohydrate loading in human muscle: an improved 1 day protocol.
Retrieved 12 27, 2012, from PubMed.gov:
http://www.ncbi.nlm.nih.gov/pubmed/12111292
ymcaed.org.uk/mus

Cahill, G. J. (1976). Starvation in man. Retrieved January 03, 2013, from
PubMed.gov: http://www.ncbi.nlm.nih.gov/pubmed/182420
ymcaed.org.uk/sta

Coggan, A. R., & Coyle, E. F. (1991). Carbohydrate ingestion during
prolonged exercise: effects on metabolism and performance. Retrieved
January 19, 2013, from PubMed.gov:
http://www.ncbi.nlm.nih.gov/pubmed/1936083
ymcaed.org.uk/cax

Coyle, E. F. (1991). Timing and method of increased carbohydrate intake to
cope with heavy training, competition and recovery. Retrieved January 02,
2013, from PubMed.gov: http://www.ncbi.nlm.nih.gov/pubmed/1895362
ymcaed.org.uk/com

Coyle, E. F. (1995). Substrate utilization during exercise in active people.
Retrieved January 02, 2013, from PubMed.gov:
http://www.ncbi.nlm.nih.gov/pubmed/7900696
ymcaed.org.uk/uti

Fairchild, T. J., et al. (2002). Rapid carbohydrate loading after a short bout
of near maximal intensity exercise. Retrieved 12 27, 2012, from

PubMed.gov: http://www.ncbi.nlm.nih.gov/pubmed/12048325
ymcaed.org.uk/bou

Fleck, S. J., & Kraemer, W. J. (1987). Designing Resistance Training Programs. Champaign, Illinois: Human Kinetics Publishers.

Ganio, M. S., Klau, J. F., Casa, D. J., Armstrong, L. E., & Maresh, C. M. (2009). Effect of caffeine on sport-specific endurance performance: a systematic review. Retrieved January 18, 2013, from PubMed.gov: http://www.ncbi.nlm.nih.gov/pubmed/19077738
ymcaed.org.uk/caf

Hoffman, J. R., & Falvo, M. J. (2004). Protein – Which is Best. Journal of Sports Science and Medicine, 3 (3): 118–30.

Lemon, P. W. (1996, April). Is increased dietary protein necessary or beneficial for individuals with a physically active lifestyle? Retrieved January 15, 2013, from PubMed.gov: http://www.ncbi.nlm.nih.gov/pubmed/8700446
ymcaed.org.uk/phy

Loucks, A. B., Kiens, B., & Wright, H. H. (2011). Energy availability in athletes. Journal of Sports Sciences, 29(S1), S7 - S15.

Phillips, S. M. (2012, August). Dietary protein requirements and adaptive advantages in athletes. Retrieved January 15, 2013, from PubMed.gov: http://www.ncbi.nlm.nih.gov/pubmed/23107527
ymcaed.org.uk/ath

Phillips, S. M., & van Loon, L. J. (2011). Dietary protein for athletes: from requirements to optimum adaptation. Journal of Sports Sciences, 29(S1) S29-S38.

Powers, S., Nelson, W. B., & Larson-Meyer, E. (2011). Antioxidant and Vitamin D supplements for athletes: sense or nonsense? Retrieved January 18, 2013, from PubMed.gov: http://www.ncbi.nlm.nih.gov/pubmed/21830999
ymcaed.org.uk/vit

Powers, M. E., Nelson, W. B., & Larson-Meyer, E. (2003). Creatine supplementation increases total body water without altering fluid distribution. Journal of Athletic Training, 38 (1): 44-50.

Schofield, W. (1985). Predicting basal metabolic rate, new standards and review of previous work. Retrieved January 03, 2013, from PubMed.gov: http://www.ncbi.nlm.nih.gov/pubmed/4044297
ymcaed.org.uk/met

Sherman, W. M., Costill, D. L., Fink, W. J., & Miller, J. (1981). Effect of exercise-diet manipulation on muscle glycogen and its subsequent utilization during performance. Retrieved December 22, 2012, from PubMed.gov: http://www.ncbi.nlm.nih.gov
ymcaed.org.uk/gly

Tang J. E., Moore, D. R., Kujbida, G. W., Tarnopolsky, M. A., & Phillips, S. M. (2009). Ingestion of whey hydrolysate, casein, or soy protein isolate: effects on mixed muscle protein synthesis at rest and following resistance exercise in young men. Retrieved January 12, 2013, from PubMed.gov: http://www.ncbi.nlm.nih.gov/pubmed/19589961
ymcaed.org.uk/res

Tarpenning, K. W. (2001). Influence of weight training exercise and modification of hormonal response on skeletal muscle growth. Retrieved January 12, 2013, from PubMed.gov: http://www.ncbi.nlm.nih.gov/pubmed/11905937
ymcaed.org.uk/hor

Wootton, S. (1990). Nutrition for Sport. London: Simon & Schuster.

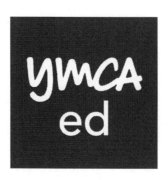

Discover more books and ebooks of interest to you and find out about the range of work we do at the forefront of health, fitness and wellbeing.

www.ymcaed.org.uk